Belly Fat Loss

22 Viable, Fundamental And Without-diet Tips To Lose Belly Fat Rapidly And Normally

By

Jane Williams

Table Of Contents

Introduction

22 vital tips on losing belly fat

Conclusion

Introduction

Can we be factual for a moment: that marshmallowy center didn't arrive for the time being. Upsetting days at the workplace, enjoying one-too-many cheat dinners, or tracking down reasons to skip a day, week, or even a month of exercises are making it simple to pack on the pounds — and making it hard or difficult to get them off.

Watching that additional garbage accumulate around your gut can put you at an expanded gamble for coronary illness, diabetes, and early passing. Fortunately, getting in shape and shedding midsection fat doesn't need to take for eternity.

For a slimmer belly, better body, and diminished hazard of ongoing illness, begin with these simple and solid tips to lose gut fat that are upheld by science.

1. Beginning Your Day Early

Try not to let additional hours relaxing in bed stand between you and a compliment stomach. While getting sufficient rest can assist with helping your metabolic rate, staying in bed might fix any advantage you'd appreciate from taking a nap. Weight study reveals that late sleepers who rested past 10:45 in the first part of the day ate almost 250 additional calories throughout the span of the day, notwithstanding eating half as many fruits and vegetables as their timely riser counterparts. Much more terrible, they chowed down on more pungent, sweet, and trans-fat-loaded inexpensive food than the individuals who got up before. In the event that you end up going away from the house early, you're in for an extra metabolic lift; individuals presented to only a brief time of early morning daylight have lower BMIs than their late-waking partners.

2. Eat More Berries Stacked With Cancer Prevention Agents

Rather than fulfilling your sweet tooth with refined sugar, go to berries and partake in a slimmer waistline in a matter of moments without working out. Berries are stacked with cell reinforcements, which can assist with decreasing irritation all through the body, and examination uncovers that rodents given a cherry-rich eating regimen shaved off a huge extent of their tummy fat when contrasted with a benchmark group. Berries like strawberries, raspberries, blueberries, and blackberries are likewise stacked with resveratrol, a cell reinforcement shade that has been connected to decreases in gut fat and a diminished gamble of dementia, for sure.

3. Keep Away From Trans Fat and Hydrogenated Oils

Those trans fats on your menu are hanging out on display and subverting your lean tummy designs each time you eat them. In the event that a food item says it contains to some extent hydrogenated oils, you're eating trans fat, which can expand your gamble of coronary illness, elevated cholesterol, and weight with each chomp. Truth be told, research directed uncovers that monkeys whose diets contained eight percent trans fat increased their muscle fat by 7.2 percent, while those who ate monounsaturated fat acquired only a small portion of that sum. Rather than allowing hurtful trans fat to occupy room on your menu, top off with these sound fats.

4.   Change to Sprouted Bread

While it's generally accepted that bread is untouchable while you're attempting to lose tummy fat, the right bread may really assist the interaction. Changing to sprouted bread can help carb-lovers anxious to get their fix without going up a belt size, because of the inulin content of grown grains. The results of a review distributed in Nourishment and Digestion uncover that pre-diabetic review subjects whose diets were enhanced with inulin shaved off more gut fat and complete load than those whose dinner plans didn't pack this solid prebiotic fiber.

5. Lift Loads

Do you try to lift? Assuming you don't joke around about disposing of that paunch fat quickly, obstruction preparing may very well be the key. Investigations discovered that adding weight lifting to grown-up male subjects' exercises fundamentally decreased their chances of stomach stoutness over a long term concentrate period, in spite of the fact that doing likewise measures of cardio made no such difference. Another Exploration even found that only four months of weight lifting supported concentrate on subjects' metabolic rates by an incredible 7.7 percent, making it simpler to dump those extra crawls around your center.

6. Quit Adding Sugars to Your Food and Beverages

While many individuals go to counterfeit sugars in an off track endeavor to shave their waistlines, those phony sugars are probably going to make the contrary difference. As per research, fake sugars are really connected with an expanded gamble of stomach corpulence and weight gain, conceivably in light of the fact that they can set off desires for the genuine stuff and spike insulin levels likewise to genuine sugar.

7. Eat More Fiber

The key to a slimmer stomach in the blink of an eye? A ton of fiber in your diet. Although many individuals are opposed to adding carbs to their eating routine while they're attempting to get in shape, adding the right, fiber-rich food varieties can assist you with decreasing paunch fat rapidly.

Here are rich-fiber varieties of food you ought to eat to lose stomach fat quick:

- Beans, peas, and lentils
- Nuts and Seeds
- Berries
- Squash
- Broccoli
- Entire Grains

As a matter of fact, research found that each 10-gram everyday expansion in solvent fiber was related with a 3.7 percent decline in perilous instinctive fat for more than five years. The people who were dynamic got even less fatty, shaving off two times that much fat in a similar measure of time. To begin dumping that additional stomach fat today, add the best high-fiber food varieties to your menu!

8. Trade Ketchup For Salsa

Without a doubt, ketchup is delicious, but on the other hand it's a significant saboteur with regards to your weight reduction endeavors. Ketchup is stacked with sugar — as much as four grams for every tablespoon — and looks similar to the natural product from which it's determined. Fortunately, trading out your ketchup for salsa can assist you with shaving off that midsection fat at home without an eating regimen. New tomatoes, similar to those utilized in salsa, are stacked with lycopene, which helps in decreases in both by and large fat and abdomen outline. Assuming you like your salsa zesty, all the better; the capsaicin in hot peppers, as jalapeños and chipotles, can help your digestion, as well.

9. Get More Vitamin D

While few would propose you fire hitting up the tanning beds for better wellbeing, getting some normal daylight can assist you with disposing of paunch fat very quickly. Research found that vitamin D-insufficient overweight ladies somewhere in the range of 50 and 75 who increased their admission of the alleged daylight nutrient shed more weight and muscle to fat ratio than the people who didn't. To rehearse safe sun, ensure you're restricting yourself to 15 sans sunscreen minutes out of every day.

10.   Eat More Nuts

Some of the time, to get your body ready, you need to get somewhat nutty. While nuts are high in fat, that exceptionally fat makes them such strong weapons in the conflict against a swelling stomach. Truth be told, a review distributed in Diabetes Care uncovered that concentrate on members who consumed an eating routine wealthy in monounsaturated fats, similar to those found in nuts, over a 28-day time frame acquired less midsection fat than their soaked fat-consuming partners while likewise further developing their insulin responsiveness.

11. Attempt an Extreme Focus Fat Consume Work-out Daily Practice

Rather than exposing yourself to one more unending exercise, wrench up the power and you'll get results quicker than you at any point expected.

These are the best activities that can assist you with losing stomach fat quick and dispose of undesirable calories:

Level link woodshop

- Sets: 2
- Reps: 10 on each side
- Rest: 60-90 sec

Deadlift

- Sets: 3-5
- Reps: 6
- Rest: 0 sec

Twisted around line

- Sets: 3-5
- Reps: 6
- Rest: 0 sec

Hang clean

- Sets: 3-5
- Reps: 6
- Rest: 0 sec

Push press

- Sets: 3-5
- Reps: 6
- Rest: 0 sec

Squats

- Sets: 4
- Reps: 5
- Rest: 0 sec

Above press

- Sets: 4
- Reps: 5
- Rest: 0 sec

Single-leg Romanian deadlift

- Sets: 4
- Reps: 5 on each side
- Rest: 0 sec

Jawline up

- Sets: 4
- Reps: 5
- Rest: 90 sec

The results of a PLOS One review uncover that grown-up male review subjects who practiced seriously briefly had comparable respiratory and metabolic changes to the individuals who worked out at a slower speed for near 60 minutes, so to consume that stomach fat, say so long to slow and steady.

12. Flavor Your Food With Garlic

A little garlic in your feasts could mean significantly less weight around your center. The outcome of a Korean report found that mice given a high-fat eating regimen enhanced with garlic lost fundamentally more weight and stomach fat than the ones who just ate greasy food sources. Far better, they likewise worked on their liver wellbeing, causing it simpler to remain solid and to consume off that overabundant fat in the long haul. For additional delightful ways of making your food more agreeable, go to the digestion supporting fiery recipes and watch those pounds dissolve away.

13. Clean Your Teeth

Keeping a toothbrush convenient can accomplish more than cleaning up that grin (and counter the impacts of all that stomach thinning garlic); cleaning your teeth over the course of the day can likewise assist you with dumping that midsection fat quickly. A review directed by an example of more than 14,000 members observed that brushing after each feast was connected to bring down weight. That minty toothpaste flavor conflicts with basically every food, except brushing may likewise set off a Pavlovian reaction that tells your mind the kitchen's shut.

14. Eat More Omega-3s With Fish

In the event that you have weight to lose and you need it gone quickly, take a stab at trading out your typical proteins for fish. Besides the fact that fish lower in is calories than a comparable measure of hamburger or chicken, however a review distributed in Corpulence additionally uncovers concentrate on subjects who added omega-3 unsaturated fats, similar to those tracked down in fish, to their eating regimens shed more weight and made some simpler memories keeping it off than the people who skipped them.

15. Keep Entire Grains in Your Eating Regimen

You don't need to go low-carb to discard those additional pounds around your midriff in a brief timeframe.

To dispose of stomach fat, ditch refined grains like white bread and white rice, and eat all the more entire grains, for example,

- Cereal
- Quinoa
- Entire wheat pasta
- Earthy colored rice
- Grain
- Farro

Truth be told, choosing all the more entire grains may very well get you there quicker. Research has connected eating at least three day to day servings of entire grains to however much a 10 percent decrease in instinctive body fat ratio, the sort that ups your chances for constant illnesses, similar to diabetes, coronary illness, and hypertension.

16. Add A few Acidic Food Sources

Try not to purchase your ticket to Bonnaroo at this time; the sort of corrosive that will assist you with thinning down is the stuff just inside your bureau. A review distributed in Bioscience, Biotechnology, and Organic chemistry uncovered that large review subjects who made vinegar some portion of their eating routine dropped more paunch fat than a benchmark group, and other exploration proposes that acidic food sources, similar to vinegar, can build the human starch digestion by as much as 40%.

17. Nibble on Veggies

Your folks weren't joking about how significant veggies are for a solid body. Everything they presumably didn't say to you, nonetheless, was that nibbling on veggies is likewise one of the simplest ways of shedding undesirable midsection fat, as well. As per a review distributed in the Diary of the Foundation of Sustenance and Dietetics, deciding on non-boring veggies, similar to cauliflower, broccoli, and cucumber, as tidbits assisted overweight children with shedding 17% of their instinctive fat while further developing their insulin responsiveness over a five-year time span.

18. Consume a Combo of Calcium and Vitamin D

Adding an additional calcium and vitamin D to your eating routine could be the most effective way to get the leveled stomach you've been dreaming about. Over only a year, research found that large female review subjects who increased their calcium consumption shed 11 pounds of fat to a large ratio without other significant dietary changes. To keep your calcium decisions solid, take a stab at stirring it up between dairy sources, calcium-rich salad greens, greasy fish, nuts, and seeds.

19. Nibble on Tart Cherries

That sharp cherry is sweet with regards to your wellbeing. The reports of a review found that rodents given high-fat food sources alongside tart cherries dumped nine percent more body fat than those in a benchmark group over only 12 weeks. Cherries are likewise a decent wellspring antioxidant pigment resveratrol, which has been connected to decreases in gut fat, dementia hazard, and lower paces of macular degeneration among the old.

20. Increase Your Cardio Exercise

You don't need to become the next Usain Bolt in the making to enjoy some serious belly-slimming results from hitting the track from time to time. Indeed, even a moderate-rate run a couple of times each week can impact through that stomach fat; as a matter of fact, an investigation discovered that, throughout the span of an eight-month study, overweight grown-up concentrate on subjects who ran 12 miles seven days lost the most tummy fat and copied 67% a greater number of calories than members who did a comparable measure of obstruction work out, or a blend of cardio and opposition work.

21. Get More Rest

Need to lose that midsection fat quick? In your fantasies! However, truly: a decent night's rest is one of the most mind-blowing ways of disposing of that additional fat around your midsection for good. Among the 60,000 ladies partaking in the Medical caretakers' Wellbeing Review, the people who rested for less than five hours a night were at the most serious gamble of becoming hefty and acquiring at least 30 pounds throughout the review period when contrasted with the people who dozed for at least seven hours.

22. Try Not To Have After Supper

Quit dealing with your kitchen like the entire night burger joint and you'll quit seeing those undesirable pounds heaping onto your casing, as well. The results of a review distributed in

Cell Digestion found that mice who just approached food during an eight-hour time frame remained thin throughout the span of the review, while those who ate a similar number of calories of a 16-hour term put on essentially more weight, especially around their center. At the point when you're done with supper around evening time, shut the cooler and don't think back until morning — your midsection will be much obliged. At the point when you really do go to the kitchen in the A.M., ensure the best solid kitchen staples for cooking are hanging tight for you.

<u>Conclusion</u>

For some individuals, lessening how much stomach fat can fundamentally work on their wellbeing. Individuals can accomplish this by taking on an empowering diet and work-out everyday practice.